Copyright © 2024

All rights reserved. No part of this publication may be reproduced, distributed, or transmitted in any form or by any means, including photocopying, recording, or other electronic or mechanical methods, without the prior written permission of the publisher, except in the case of brief quotations embodied in critical reviews and certain other noncommercial uses permitted by copyright law

Unseen Struggle

Navigating the Complex World of Chronic Fatigue Syndrome

Contents

Introduction 5
Chapter 1: What is Chronic Fatigue Syndrome? 6
    Definition and Symptoms 6
    How It Differs from Ordinary Fatigue 7
Chapter 2: The Causes of CFS 8
    Possible Viral Links 8
    Genetic Factors 8
    Environmental Triggers 9
    Other Theories 9
Chapter 3: Diagnosing CFS 10
    Challenges in Diagnosis 10
    Criteria and Medical Tests 10
    Emerging Tools and Biomarkers 11
Chapter 4: Living with CFS 12
    Daily Impact 12
    Personal Stories 13
    Strategies for Managing Day-to-Day Life 13
Chapter 5: Treatment and Management 14
    Current Treatment Approaches 14
    Lifestyle and Home Remedies 15
    Environmental Modifications: 15
    Role of Diet and Exercise 15

    Considerations for Long-Term Management 16
Chapter 6: Psychological Effects 17
    Mental Health Challenges 17
    Coping Mechanisms 17
    Importance of Holistic Care 18
Chapter 7: Research and Hope 19
    Recent Advances in Research 19
    Future Prospects 20
Chapter 8: Supporting Someone with CFS 21
    How Families and Friends Can Help 21
    Resources and Support Networks 22
Conclusion 23

Introduction

Chronic Fatigue Syndrome (CFS) is a complex, often misunderstood illness that affects millions worldwide. Commonly characterized by extreme fatigue that doesn't improve with rest and can be worsened by physical or mental activity, CFS poses a significant challenge not only to those who suffer from it but also to the medical community that seeks to understand it. This illness, often invisible to the naked eye, impacts the lives of patients significantly, influencing their ability to perform everyday tasks that many take for granted.

In this guide we delve into the nuances of this enigmatic condition. The aim is to shed light on what it means to live with CFS, the science behind its diagnosis, and the current options for management and treatment. We will explore the various theories about the causes of CFS, from viral infections to genetic predisposition, and consider the environmental triggers that may precipitate its onset.

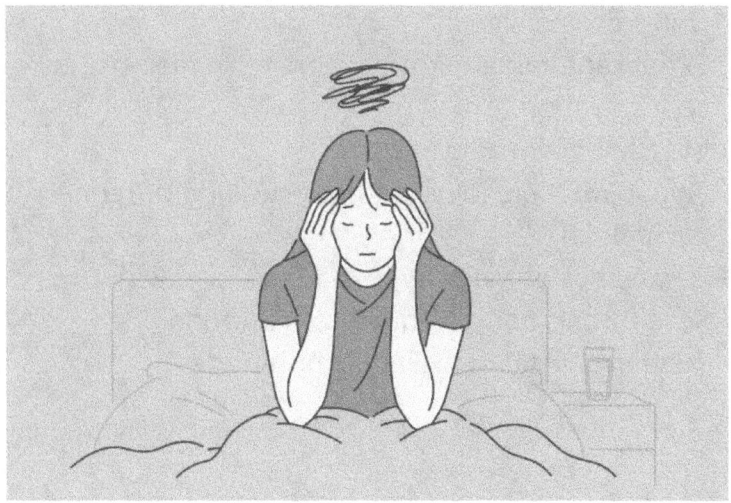

Chapter 1: What is Chronic Fatigue Syndrome?

Chronic Fatigue Syndrome (CFS), also known as Myalgic Encephalomyelitis (ME), is a debilitating disorder characterized by profound tiredness or fatigue that is not improved by rest and is not directly caused by other medical conditions. The fatigue significantly interferes with daily activities and work, which makes it a major cause of disability.

Definition and Symptoms

CFS is more than just regular tiredness. The fatigue experienced by those with CFS is severe, persistent, and can dramatically limit their functional capacity. According to criteria developed by medical professionals, for a diagnosis of CFS to be considered, this incapacitating fatigue must be present for at least six months and must be accompanied by at least four out of the following eight symptoms:

- Post-exertional malaise lasting more than 24 hours.
- Unrefreshing sleep.
- Significant impairment of short-term memory or concentration.
- Muscle pain (myalgia).
- Pain in multiple joints without swelling or redness (arthralgia).
- Headaches of a new type, pattern, or severity.
- Sore throat that is frequent or recurring.
- Tender cervical or axillary lymph nodes.

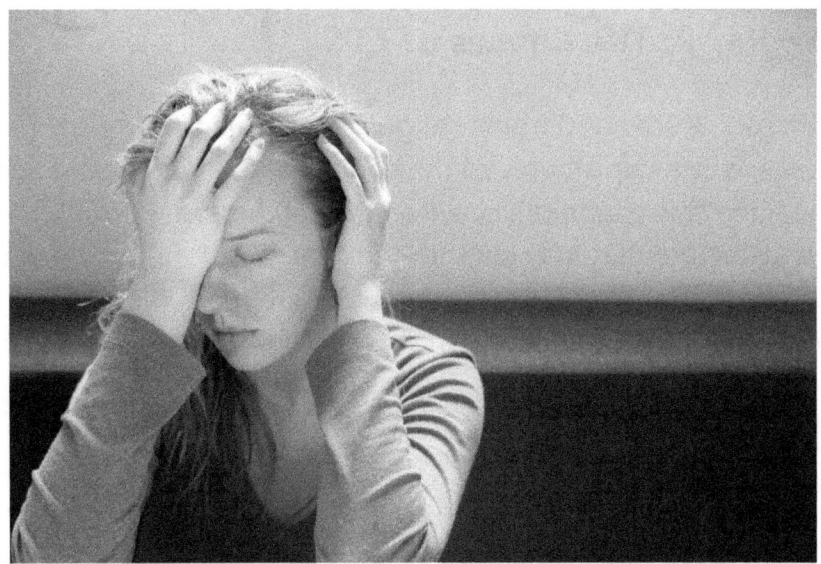

These symptoms must not have pre-existed the fatigue and must not abate with rest. This criterion underscores the chronic, unyielding nature of the syndrome and helps differentiate it from other conditions that might cause similar symptoms.

How It Differs from Ordinary Fatigue

Unlike typical fatigue that people experience after physical exertion or a busy day, the fatigue associated with CFS does not arise from excessive recent activity and disproportionately disrupts normal activities. Moreover, CFS fatigue does not resolve with rest or sleep, which is often restorative in other forms of fatigue.

The key differentiator in CFS is post-exertional malaise (PEM), a worsening of symptoms following even minor physical or mental exertion. This response is unique and pivotal for diagnosis, as it highlights the body's inability to recover after expending even small amounts of energy.

Chapter 2: The Causes of CFS

The exact causes of Chronic Fatigue Syndrome (CFS) remain elusive, which contributes to the complexity of diagnosing and managing this condition. However, researchers have identified several factors that may contribute to the development of CFS. These include viral infections, immune system problems, hormonal imbalances, and genetic predisposition.

Possible Viral Links

One of the earliest and most examined theories is that certain viral infections may trigger CFS. Historically, outbreaks of CFS have been associated with epidemics of particular viruses. For example, a significant number of CFS cases were reported following infection with the Epstein-Barr virus, a common cause of mononucleosis. Other viral links include human herpesvirus 6, enterovirus, and possibly the recently highlighted coronavirus (as post-viral fatigue syndromes are observed in COVID-19 survivors).

Researchers hypothesize that these viruses may trigger an abnormal immune response or cause lasting damage to the immune system, which in turn leads to the symptoms of CFS. However, not everyone who gets infected with these viruses develops CFS, suggesting that other factors are also at play.

Genetic Factors

Genetics may also play a role in CFS. Studies have found that the condition appears more frequently in some families, and certain genetic markers are associated with an increased risk of developing the syndrome. This familial clustering suggests that genetic predisposition could influence an individual's susceptibility to CFS, possibly affecting the immune system's response to triggers.

Environmental Triggers

Environmental factors are another area of interest. Physical or emotional stress, such as a traumatic event or serious injury, can precede the onset of CFS symptoms. Additionally, people who experience severe, prolonged stress may be more vulnerable to developing the condition. Other environmental contributors could include exposure to toxins or pollutants, which are hypothesized to affect the central nervous system and immune function.

Other Theories

Some researchers are exploring the possibility that an imbalance in the gut microbiome or a dysregulation of the nervous system could contribute to CFS. There is also investigation into the role of mitochondrial dysfunction, where cells do not produce energy efficiently, leading to the profound fatigue characteristic of CFS.

Chapter 3: Diagnosing CFS

Diagnosing Chronic Fatigue Syndrome (CFS) is a challenging process. There are no specific tests that can definitively diagnose CFS, and its symptoms overlap with many other medical conditions. Therefore, the diagnosis is largely based on exclusion and careful consideration of clinical criteria.

Challenges in Diagnosis

One of the primary challenges in diagnosing CFS is the absence of a universal diagnostic test. Health professionals must rely on patient histories, symptom checklists, and physical exams to make their assessments. This process often requires ruling out other conditions that could explain the symptoms, such as sleep disorders, mental health issues, autoimmune diseases, and hormonal imbalances. This necessitates a series of tests to exclude these other conditions, which can be time-consuming and frustrating for patients.

Criteria and Medical Tests

The most widely accepted criteria for diagnosing CFS come from the Centers for Disease Control and Prevention (CDC), which focus on the presence of unexplained persistent fatigue that is not improved by rest, lasts for at least six months, and is accompanied by four or more of the additional symptoms listed in Chapter 1.

In addition to using these criteria, doctors may perform various tests to rule out other conditions:

- Blood tests: These can check for anemia, thyroid problems, and signs of infection.
- Sleep studies: To exclude sleep disorders that could cause fatigue.
- Immune system tests: Looking for markers of inflammation or other immune abnormalities.
- Mental health evaluations: To assess whether depression or anxiety might be contributing to the fatigue.

Despite these tools, the diagnosis of CFS often remains one of exclusion. The subjectivity involved in evaluating symptoms and the variety of symptoms that can be present make the diagnostic process complex.

Emerging Tools and Biomarkers

Researchers are working to identify biomarkers and develop tests that could more clearly diagnose CFS. Studies into immune system changes, energy metabolism, and brain function offer promising avenues. For instance, some researchers are investigating whether certain patterns in cytokines (proteins involved in cell signaling in the immune system) or abnormalities in MRI brain scans could serve as diagnostic tools.

Until such tools are validated and widely available, the medical community must rely on a combination of patient history, symptom tracking, and exclusion of other diseases to diagnose CFS. This approach underscores the necessity for a thorough and empathetic understanding from healthcare providers to manage and treat CFS effectively.

Chapter 4: Living with CFS

Living with Chronic Fatigue Syndrome (CFS) presents unique challenges. The invisible nature of the illness often leads to misunderstandings and stigma, complicating both personal relationships and professional life. This chapter explores the daily impact of CFS and shares personal stories from those navigating life with this condition.

Daily Impact

The pervasive fatigue associated with CFS can profoundly affect every aspect of daily life. Simple tasks such as showering, cooking, or even communicating can become overwhelmingly exhausting. The unpredictability of symptom flare-ups further complicates planning and activities, leading many sufferers to reduce or give up their hobbies and social activities.

Physical Limitations: Physical activities need to be carefully managed to avoid post-exertional malaise, a hallmark symptom of CFS. This often requires patients to pace themselves, breaking tasks into smaller steps with rest periods in between.

Cognitive Challenges: Known as "brain fog" among the CFS community, cognitive impairments include difficulties with memory, concentration, and information processing. This can affect personal relationships, academic performance, and professional responsibilities.

Emotional and Social Effects: The isolation that comes from living with a misunderstood illness can lead to feelings of loneliness, frustration, and depression. The lack of visible symptoms can cause disbelief or skepticism from friends, family, and even medical professionals, further isolating those affected.

Personal Stories

Emily's Story: Emily was a high school teacher whose life changed drastically after developing CFS. Despite her active and social lifestyle, Emily now finds herself managing her energy like a limited currency, choosing between everyday activities and conserving energy for her work. The skepticism she faces from colleagues who don't understand why she looks "fine" but can't engage as before has been one of her toughest battles.

Mark's Story: Mark was an avid runner before CFS took its toll. Now, he focuses on small, manageable walks and uses mindfulness techniques to cope with the frustration of not being able to engage in intense physical activity. His journey has been one of acceptance, learning to value what he can do rather than mourning his past capabilities.

Strategies for Managing Day-to-Day Life

Pacing: A key strategy for managing CFS is pacing, which involves balancing activity and rest to avoid exacerbating symptoms. This may mean setting incremental goals and gradually increasing activity levels without overdoing it.

Support Systems: Building a supportive network, including healthcare providers who understand CFS, is crucial. Support groups, whether online or in-person, can also provide a sense of community and mutual understanding.

Adaptations at Home and Work: Many find that making adjustments at home and work can help manage symptoms. This might include flexible working hours, working from home, or ergonomic adjustments to reduce physical strain.

Chapter 5: Treatment and Management

While there is no cure for Chronic Fatigue Syndrome (CFS), there are various treatment strategies that can help manage symptoms and improve quality of life. This chapter explores current treatment approaches, lifestyle modifications, and the role of diet and exercise in managing CFS.

Current Treatment Approaches

Medical Treatments:

- Antiviral medications: For some patients, particularly those whose CFS may be linked to viral infections, antiviral medications can provide relief.
- Immunomodulators: These drugs, which alter the immune system's functioning, are being explored for their potential benefits in CFS patients who exhibit immune system abnormalities.
- Pain relief medications: Non-steroidal anti-inflammatory drugs (NSAIDs) and other pain relievers can be used to manage joint and muscle pain associated with CFS.
- Sleep aids: Medications to help regulate sleep patterns can be critical, as restorative sleep is often a major challenge for those with CFS.

Therapeutic Treatments:

- Cognitive Behavioral Therapy (CBT): This psychological intervention helps patients cope with the condition by changing negative thought patterns and behaviors.
- Graded Exercise Therapy (GET): Initially controversial, GET involves a structured increase in physical activity to

gradually raise the patient's tolerance. This must be tailored to each individual's capabilities to avoid exacerbating symptoms.
- Pacing Therapy: This strategy teaches patients to balance rest and activity to prevent post-exertional malaise.

Lifestyle and Home Remedies

Dietary Adjustments:

- Many patients find symptom relief through dietary changes. This can include eliminating potential allergens like gluten or dairy, reducing sugar intake, and increasing hydration.
- Supplements: Some find benefits from supplements such as Vitamin B12, magnesium, and omega-3 fatty acids, though these should be used under the guidance of a healthcare provider.

Environmental Modifications:

- Creating a restful environment at home, reducing noise and light during rest periods, and using ergonomic furniture can help alleviate symptoms.
- Managing stress through meditation, yoga, or tai chi can also be beneficial, as stress exacerbation is a common trigger for symptom flare-ups.

Role of Diet and Exercise

The relationship between diet, exercise, and CFS is complex. While no specific diet is prescribed for CFS, many patients report feeling better with balanced, nutrient-rich meals.

Similarly, exercise must be approached carefully; too much can lead to relapses, but appropriate, gentle exercise may improve overall health and energy levels.

Considerations for Long-Term Management

Living with CFS requires adapting to the chronic nature of the illness, which includes regular consultations with healthcare providers to monitor symptoms and adapt treatment plans as needed. It also involves educating friends and family about the condition to ensure supportive relationships.

The goal of treatment and management is not necessarily to eliminate symptoms but to improve functional capacity and enhance quality of life. By employing a combination of medical treatment, lifestyle adjustments, and supportive therapies, those with CFS can hope to achieve better health outcomes and a greater degree of normalcy in their daily lives.

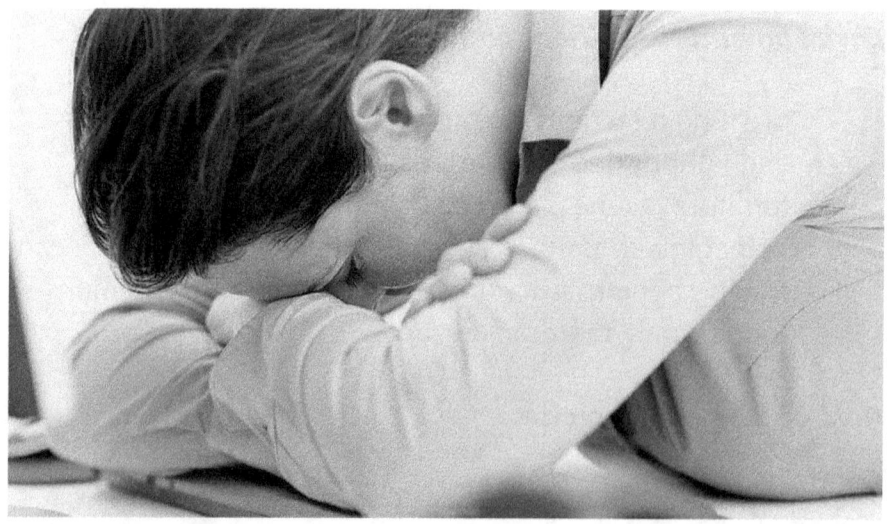

Chapter 6: Psychological Effects

Chronic Fatigue Syndrome (CFS) affects more than just the physical body; it also has profound psychological impacts.

Mental Health Challenges

Depression and Anxiety: A significant number of individuals with CFS also experience symptoms of depression and anxiety. The relentless nature of fatigue, the uncertainty of symptom flare-ups, and the overall decrease in quality of life can lead to feelings of helplessness and hopelessness, common precursors to depression. Anxiety can stem from the worry about the unpredictability of symptoms and the stress of managing a chronic condition.

Isolation and Loneliness: Due to the misunderstood nature of CFS, sufferers often feel isolated from their peers. The inability to engage in regular social activities or maintain a normal work schedule can lead to loneliness and a sense of being disconnected from others.

Stigma and Misunderstanding: CFS is frequently mischaracterized as a psychological ailment rather than a physiological one, which can lead to stigma from both the public and medical professionals. This misunderstanding can exacerbate the emotional distress of those with the condition.

Coping Mechanisms

Cognitive Behavioral Therapy (CBT): CBT has been shown to be effective in helping patients manage the psychological aspects of chronic illnesses, including CFS. By addressing negative thought patterns and promoting more adaptive behaviors and coping strategies, CBT can alleviate symptoms of depression and anxiety.

Support Groups: Engaging with support groups, either in person or online, can provide a network of understanding and support. These groups offer a platform for sharing experiences and strategies for coping with CFS, reducing feelings of isolation.

Mindfulness and Relaxation Techniques: Practices such as mindfulness meditation, progressive muscle relaxation, and guided imagery can help reduce stress and improve emotional well-being. These techniques also aid in managing pain and fatigue by promoting a state of relaxation and increased body awareness.

Regular Medical Follow-up: Maintaining regular contact with healthcare providers can help manage the psychological aspects of CFS. Healthcare professionals can provide not only medical treatment but also support and validation, which are crucial for mental health.

Importance of Holistic Care

Addressing the psychological effects of CFS is as important as treating the physical symptoms. Holistic care that includes mental health support can lead to better overall health outcomes and improved quality of life. Healthcare providers should encourage patients to

Chapter 7: Research and Hope

As Chronic Fatigue Syndrome (CFS) continues to be a challenging and often misunderstood condition, ongoing research is crucial for advancing understanding and improving treatment options.

Recent Advances in Research

Immunological Discoveries: Recent studies have begun to shed light on the immunological aspects of CFS. Researchers have found abnormalities in immune system functioning in CFS patients, such as altered levels of cytokines, which are proteins involved in cell signaling that can influence the body's immune response. These findings suggest that immune dysfunction may play a role in the symptomatology of CFS, offering a potential target for new therapeutic approaches.

Genetic Research: Advances in genetic research have identified possible genetic markers that could predispose individuals to CFS. Understanding these genetic factors may help in developing personalized medicine approaches tailored to the specific biological pathways affected in different individuals.

Metabolic Studies: Studies on the metabolic changes in CFS patients are uncovering potential anomalies in energy production. Some researchers believe that mitochondrial dysfunction, where cells do not produce energy efficiently, could be a key factor in the development of fatigue. These insights are leading to investigations into metabolic supplements and treatments that could enhance cellular energy production.

Neurological Research: There is also growing evidence that CFS has a neurological component. Research using advanced imaging techniques has revealed differences in brain anatomy and function in patients with CFS. These studies are crucial for understanding the brain's role in CFS and could lead to neurologically focused treatments.

Future Prospects

Biomarker Development: One of the most promising areas of CFS research is the development of biomarkers. Biomarkers are biological indicators, typically measured in blood or other body fluids, that can signify disease states. Identifying reliable biomarkers for CFS would greatly aid in diagnosis and could also provide new targets for therapeutic intervention.

Treatment Trials: Clinical trials for new treatments, including pharmaceuticals and dietary supplements, are ongoing. These trials are essential for determining the efficacy and safety of potential new therapies that could improve quality of life for CFS patients.

Interdisciplinary Approaches: The future of CFS treatment may lie in interdisciplinary approaches that combine immunology, genetics, neurology, and metabolic science. Such approaches can provide a more comprehensive understanding and management strategy for CFS, tailored to the individual patient.

Increased Awareness and Funding: As research progresses, increased awareness and funding are vital. Greater understanding can lead to more research dollars and better healthcare provider education, ultimately benefiting those who live with CFS.

Chapter 8: Supporting Someone with CFS

Supporting someone with Chronic Fatigue Syndrome (CFS) is crucial for their well-being. This chapter provides guidance on how families, friends, and caregivers can assist someone living with CFS, along with resources and support networks that can be beneficial.

How Families and Friends Can Help

Understanding and Acceptance:

Educate Yourself: The first step in providing support is to understand what CFS is and what it is not. Learning about the symptoms, treatment options, and the nature of the illness can help supporters empathize and provide appropriate support.

Listen Actively: Allow the person with CFS to share their feelings and experiences without judgment. Recognize that their symptoms, especially fatigue, are real and debilitating.

Practical Support:

Assist with Daily Tasks: Help with household chores, errands, and other tasks to reduce their workload. This can help conserve their energy and reduce stress.

Accompany to Appointments: Offer to drive them to medical appointments or provide company if they request it, which can also help in understanding their health care regimen and progress.

Emotional Support:

Encourage Social Interaction: Help them maintain social contacts even if they can't participate in many activities. Small, quiet gatherings can be less taxing.

Be Patient: Symptoms of CFS can fluctuate and may be unpredictable. Patience is key in understanding their varying abilities from day to day.

Resources and Support Networks

Local and Online Support Groups:

Joining support groups can be helpful for both patients and caregivers. These groups provide a platform to exchange information, share experiences, and receive emotional support from others who understand the challenges of living with CFS.

Educational Materials and Workshops:

Many organizations offer educational resources that can help patients and their supporters understand the illness better and keep up to date on new research and treatments. Workshops can also teach coping and management skills tailored to the needs of CFS patients.

Mental Health Professionals:

Professional counselors or therapists, especially those familiar with chronic illness management, can be invaluable in helping manage the emotional and psychological toll of CFS on both the patient and their family.

Advocacy Groups:

Groups that advocate for CFS patients can provide updates on policy changes, insurance issues, and advocacy opportunities, which can be crucial for accessing services and improving conditions for CFS sufferers.

Conclusion

Chronic Fatigue Syndrome (CFS) is a complex, often debilitating condition that affects millions of individuals worldwide. Throughout this book, "Chronic Fatigue Syndrome: The Invisible Illness," we have explored the multifaceted nature of CFS, from its symptoms and potential causes to the challenges of diagnosis and the various treatment and management strategies available.

We have seen that CFS is more than just extreme tiredness; it is a serious chronic illness that impacts every aspect of a person's life—physical, cognitive, and emotional. The uncertainty and invisibility of the condition can lead to misunderstanding and stigma, making compassionate understanding and support from family, friends, and medical professionals critical.

Key Takeaways:

Diagnosis is Challenging: CFS is diagnosed through exclusion, requiring thorough evaluation to rule out other causes of fatigue. This process emphasizes the need for patient and meticulous assessment by healthcare providers.

Management is Multifaceted: Effective management of CFS involves a combination of medical treatment, psychological support, and lifestyle adjustments. Each patient's management plan should be tailored to their specific symptoms and circumstances.

Support is Essential: The role of family, friends, and support networks is invaluable. Understanding and empathy from loved ones and the community help mitigate the isolation that many with CFS feel.

Research Offers Hope: Ongoing research into the immunological, genetic, and metabolic aspects of CFS holds promise for better diagnostic tools and more effective treatments in the future. This research is critical to unfolding the mysteries of CFS and improving patient care.

As we move forward, it is crucial for the medical community, researchers, and the public to continue to strive for a deeper understanding of Chronic Fatigue Syndrome. Increased awareness and education about CFS will lead to better outcomes for those affected by the disease. Let us all advocate for those living with CFS, ensuring they receive the recognition and support they need to manage their condition and improve their quality of life.

By fostering a broader understanding and a supportive environment, we can help illuminate this invisible illness, bringing hope and improved care to those who live with its challenges every day.

www.ingramcontent.com/pod-product-compliance
Lightning Source LLC
Chambersburg PA
CBHW071002220526
45471CB00007B/3146